YOSHI is
YOSHI goes
Yoshi has

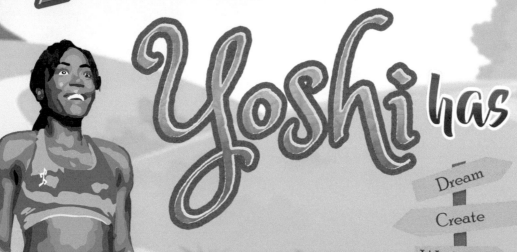

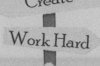

Dream

Create

Work Hard

Success

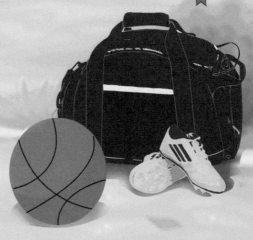

By: Yoshi Barnes

AuthorHouse™
1663 Liberty Drive
Bloomington, IN 47403
www.authorhouse.com
Phone: 1 (800) 839-8640

Published by AuthorHouse 08/30/2019

ISBN: 978-1-5462-6581-8 (sc)
ISBN: 978-1-5462-6580-1 (e)

Print information available on the last page.

Any people depicted in stock imagery provided by Getty Images are models, and such images are being used for illustrative purposes only. Certain stock imagery © Getty Images.

This book is printed on acid-free paper.

authorHOUSE®

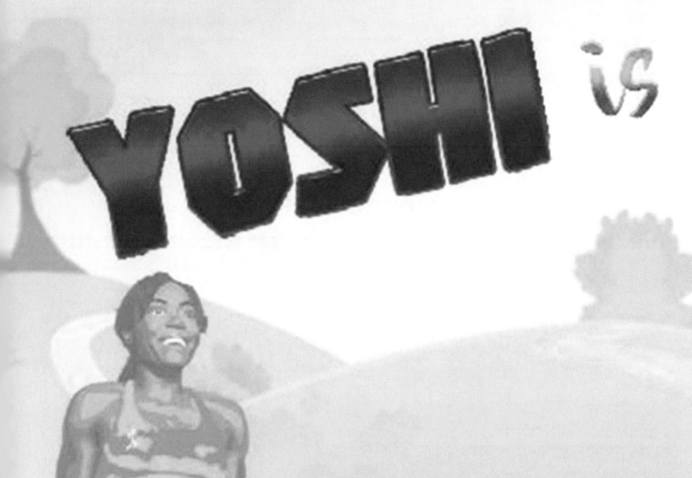

YOSHI IS THE QUEEN OF FIT. Yoshi is fast and real quick! Yoshi jumps high and big. She's strong, solid, and loves the kids. She would like you all to join in. We are headed on a Fitness Journey. Let's take a trip.

Are you ready? LET'S GO!
Yoshi has 20 jumping jacks then after that you all must lay down flat.

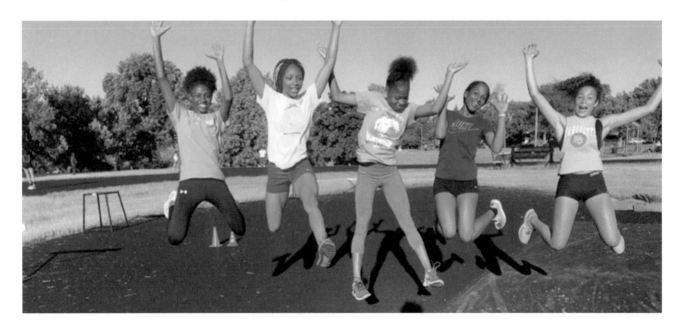

READY, SET, GO...

Yoshi has made her way through because she worked hard but so did you!

Thanks kids! Hi fives all around!

Almost to my destination!
Get ready guys and push your way through, with 10
push-ups and at the end give a WOO HOO!!

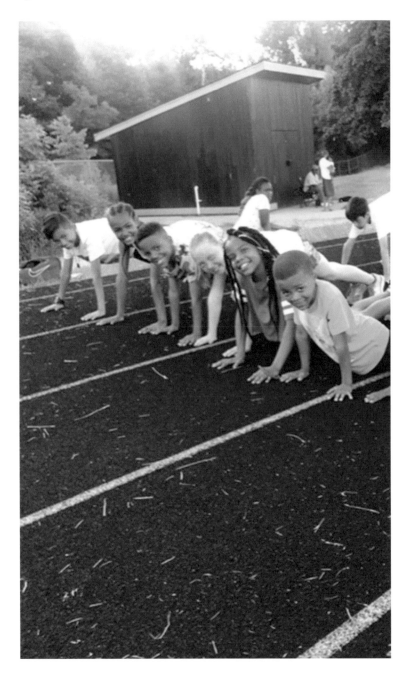

READY, SET, GO......

Awesome! You all are doing such good jobs and the last thing we have is 15 bunny hops.

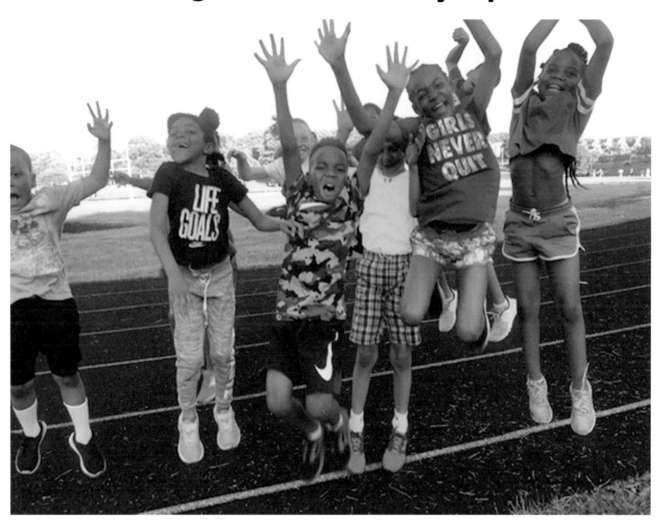

READY, SET, GO......

Let's finish our fit journey and get the things we want.

A healthy mind

A healthy body

And a healthy heart

Thanks kids! Yoshi loves journeys and would like to take you with. Yoshi is going on another trip.

ARE YOU GOING?

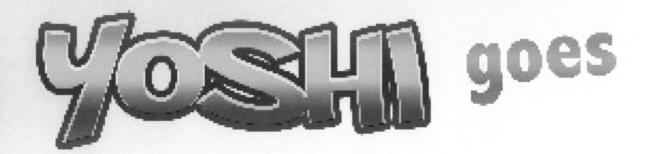

YOSHI goes

Yoshi goes to college plays basketball and runs track too. She wants to take you guys to practice to run and shoot. We have 15 jump shots.

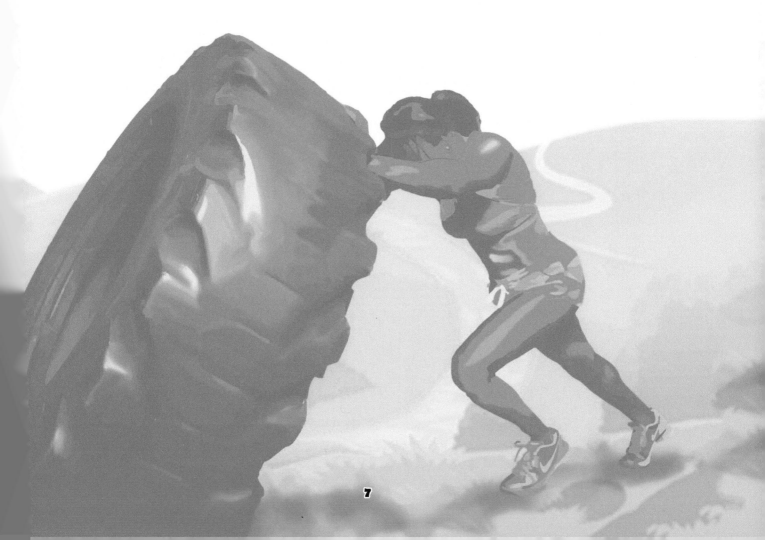

READY, SET, GO.....

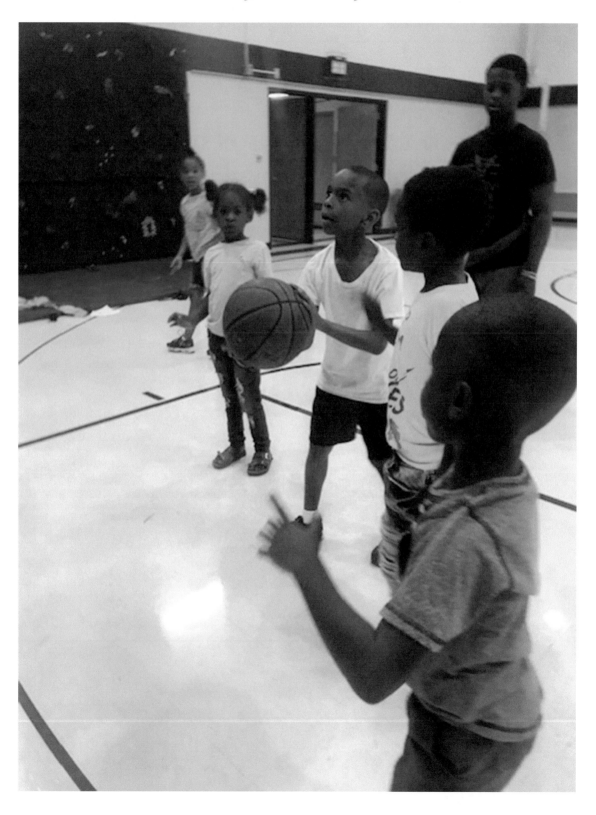

Sweet! You guys have got some good shots. Now find a space and run in the same spot.
You have 30 seconds to run in place. Go fast like you are trying to win a race.

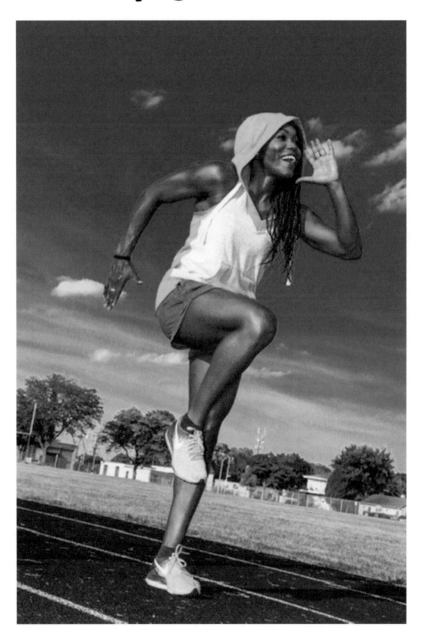

READY, SET, GO......

Nice! My heart is beating fast and I'm sweating too. That's great, it just means your body likes it and should run 30 more seconds through. It's good for practice to make sure you have it and you are fast enough to see your dreams, go grab it.

Nice! That looks really good!
Yoshi goes to training class and learns about healthy foods that help her ABS. It helps her back stay safe and will help the body last.
Now do you want to join Yoshi on this tummy task?
We have 20 sit-ups. Let's count them out loud and have a blast!

READY, SET, GO.....

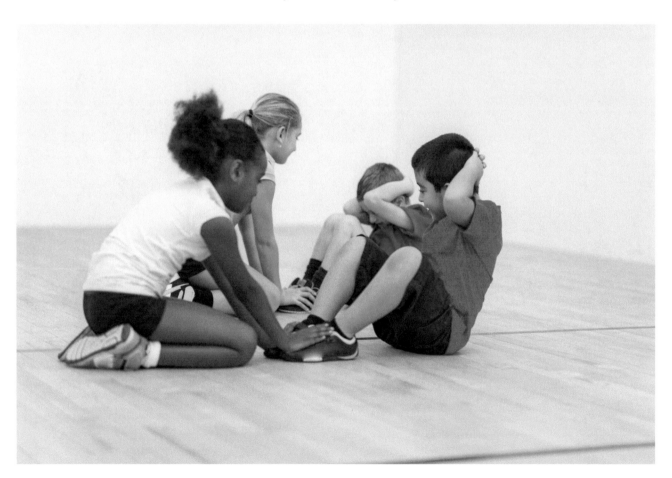

You are amazing!!
Yoshi goes to her last stop, to workout with the kids for fun and have fitness group shops. But there's one more challenge that Yoshi goes through and she really, really, really needs you. You ready? We have to count up to 30 seconds in a plank. We don't bend and we don't break!

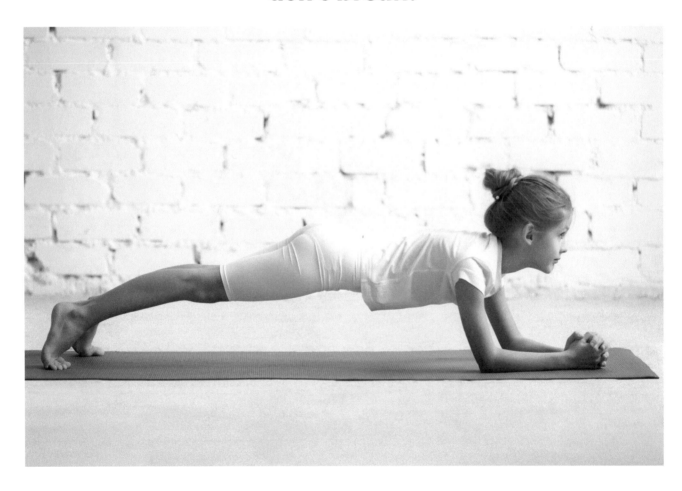

READY, SET, GO......

If your belly burns put your hands in the air and wave them side to side like you do care! You care about your health, you care about your dreams, and you care about being a decent human being.

That was fun and Yoshi really enjoys you. Thanks for helping her and yourself push through.

Yoshi loves journeys and would like to take you with. Yoshi is going on another trip....

ARE YOU GOING?

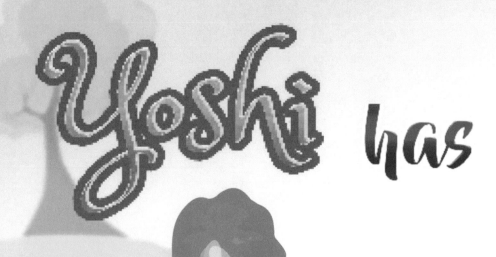

Yoshi has

Yoshi has big dreams. She really believes you can grow up and be anything.

It starts with a plan and it lives in your heart and going to school helps you stay smart. Ready for a challenge? I have 5-inch worms, 5 mountain climbers, and 5 push-ups. This will help us count. We will add it up at the end to check the amount!

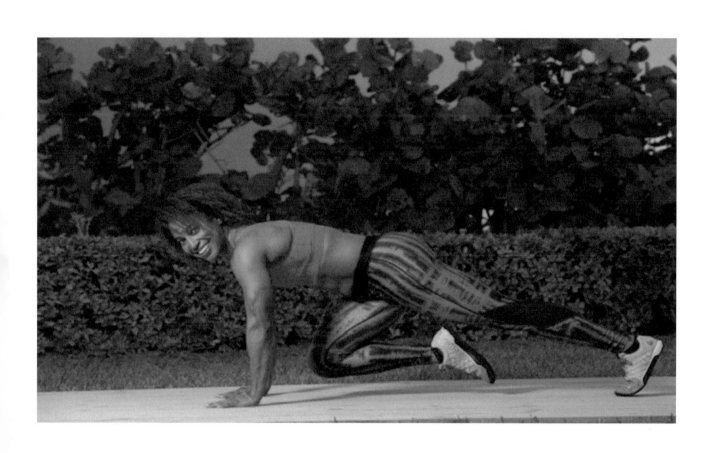

READY, SET, GO......

Sweet! What did we get? 15! How cool is that!

Yoshi has hard times just like you but if you stay positive you will always stay in good pursuits. Bad things are there to help make you stronger, to make you better, and live longer. Exercising helps with all of that so let's do 25 floor jumping jacks.

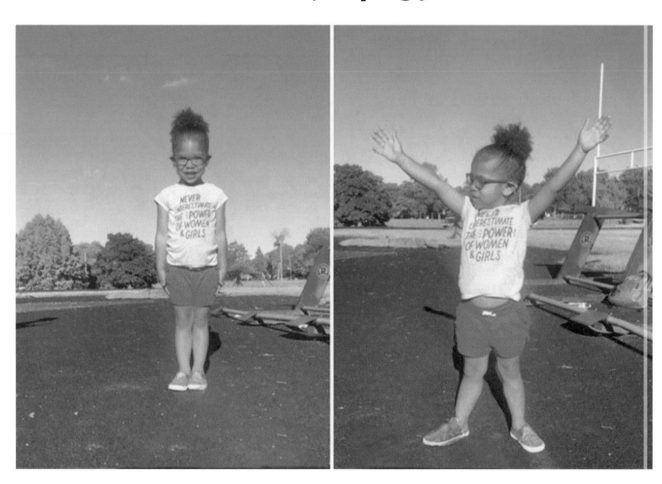

READY, SET, GO......

That was a lot. We kept going and we survived. Working hard practicing our best lives!

Thanks guys for helping Yoshi with all that she has. With your help she's able to chill and relax.
Join her one last time. We relax, lay down and enjoy our minds. Think of anything you want to be, believe that it is possible, with hard work you are unstoppable.

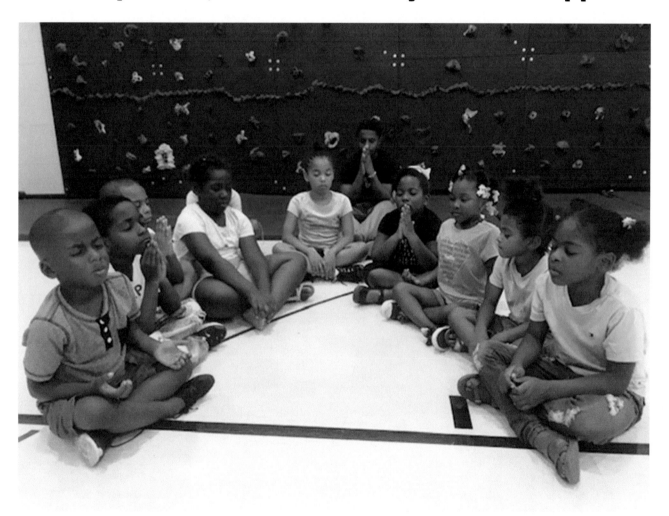

READY, SET, GO......

It's important to reflect on how hard you worked. Embrace your dreams, go after your goals, until you get a hold. Fitness is here to help with that mode. Enjoy your rest until Yoshi's next trip. Start building yours and who's coming with. ♥ ♥ ♥

Now you all are Kings and Queens of Fit! Thanks guys! Yoshi loves journeys and is super glad you came!

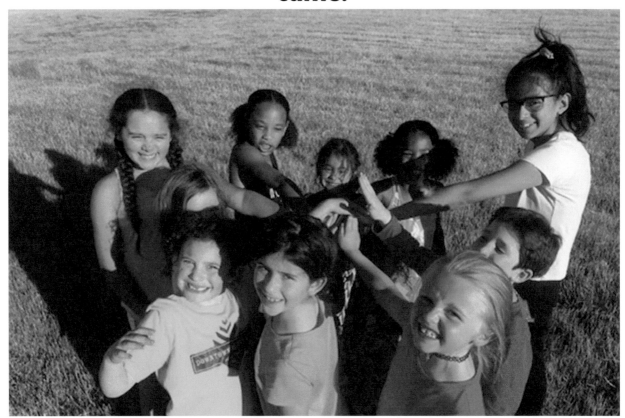

THIS HAS BEEN ONE GREAT TRIP!

THE END

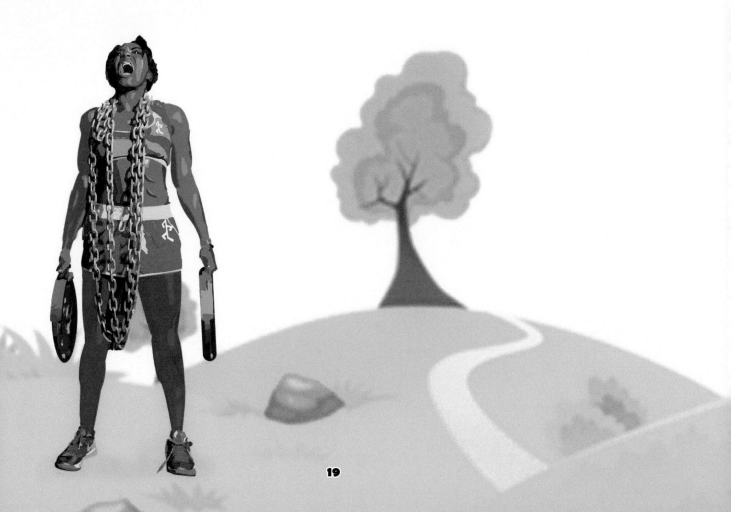

THANK YOU

First and foremost, I would like to give all glory and thanks to God. He is my reason for every thought and reasoning for being. Secondly, I'd like to thank the person reading, supporting or sharing this book. Other people are the reason my dreams of being an author is possible. Thank you for helping me fulfill my purpose.

I want to thank my family for their enduring support and belief in me. Our experiences together have shaped who I am, encouraged me, and allowed me to express who I am with the world. Thank you, Mom (Loretta Barnes) and Dad (Marcus Barnes), for always listening and being my book of wisdom. I love and appreciate you both so much.

To my editor, illustrator, graphic designer, family, and mentor Breon Worthy. Every step of the way you have guided me, pushed me, and supported my dream. One of the most valuable things you gave me was your time and attention to making this come to life. Thank you for your willingness and allowing God to be a vessel in my life.

To those who inspired me to do more, to be better, and to share God's gift THANK YOU. I value you and love you very much. (Jill Hanson, Brenda Dillard, Leah Sealey, Nicole Fernhaber, Kristin Ludwig, and many others)

Yoshi Barnes

Printed in the United States
By Bookmasters